Ayurveda Weight Loss

The Ultimate Guide to Successful Ayurvedic Detox and Weight Loss

By Michael Cesar

Table of Contents

Introduction

I want to thank you and congratulate you for buying this book, Ayurveda Weight Loss: The Ultimate Guide to Successful Ayurvedic Detox and Weight Loss. Within these pages, you will learn about the ancient and highly effective process called Ayurveda and how it relates to weight loss and the detoxification of your body.

On a daily basis, our bodies are exposed to toxins, pollution, and unhealthy dietary choices that, when combined with one another, are a time bomb just waiting to go off. The aggregate result is weight gain and difficulty removing the unwanted pounds. Toxins and unhealthy eating alone have been known to increase risks of diabetes, cancer, coronary disease, respiratory, and circulatory systems. In other words, without a healthy, safe, and effective alternative, our life span is at risk of becoming unnecessarily shortened.

This book contains proven steps and strategies on how to:

- Identify toxin exposures
- Learn about Ayurveda
- Use Ayurveda to detoxify the body and clear the mind and lose weight
- Use Ayurveda techniques to improve health and lose weight
- Make healthy choices a lifestyle, not a fad

There are plenty of reasons why ancient techniques are still being used today and the primary reason is that they work. What you're about to embark upon is a journey of recovery—a journey to recover your physical and mental health and to do so in a safe and positive environment. Weight loss fads come and go (remember the ThighMaster?), but the practice of Ayurveda has been with us for three millennia and it isn't going away any time soon. When you lose weight through Ayurveda, the weight stays off as long as you like—as long as you're adhering to your Ayurveda lifestyle.

Ayurveda Weight Loss: The Ultimate Guide to Successful Ayurvedic Detox and Weight Loss will teach you techniques that you can enjoy with your family and friends and collectively, lose weight as individuals and as a whole. Ayurveda is so effective you will be compelled to share it with those within your sphere of influence.

As with any technique for weight loss, it is important that you contact your primary care physician and talk to him/her about your plans.

Thanks again for buying Ayurveda Weight Loss: The Ultimate Guide to Successful Ayurvedic Detox and Weight Loss. I know you will enjoy it!

Chapter 1: All About Ayurveda

There are some traditions and sayings that are fundamentally timeless such as a good work ethic, early to bed and early to rise, taking time to smell the roses, loving and being loved openly, family gatherings, and adult beverages on Super Bowl Sunday. These things don't necessarily define us, but they are benchmarks, significant moments in life that shape how we see ourselves and how others see us. We cherish these moments in our history, adopt them and pass them along to our children.

The same can be said for detoxification and weight loss through Ayurveda.

Ayurveda has been around for approximately 5,000 years and has been passed down from generation to generation and the principles of Ayurveda are not only timeless, but they are effective as well. Ayurveda means "the science of life."

Ayur = Life

Veda = Science

Ayurveda has been a part of the Indian culture throughout history and is being increasingly accepted as an alternative medicine in Western culture. As mentioned in the introduction of this book, it is more than just finding a way to cure illness, it provides the human existence with a means to maintain vitality and to reach the pinnacle of human potential. It teaches that health is predicated on balance—the balance of mind, body, and spirit—not just to treat disease or infirmities. Its goal is to focus on the healthy aspects of life, rather than just eliminating the negative. When this is accomplished, the result is healthy weight loss.

This is where it may get a little complex, but stay with it and you will begin to see how Ayurveda is an amazing tradition to help detox the body and lose weight in a healthy, productive manner.

Ayurveda teaches that each of us are made of five elements in the universe:

Air, Fire, Water, Earth, Space

These five elements intertwine with each other in the human existence to create energies called "doshas." These doshas control how your body functions within its environment. The three doshas are:

Vata (air and space)

Pitta (water and fire)

Kapha (water and earth)

Every human is born with a mix of these doshas, however, one is usually more dominant than others and knowing what that may be can help in the process of losing weight through Ayurveda. The Vata dosha controls your most base bodily functions such as breathing, blood flow, heart operation, and processing waste. The Pitta dosha controls your metabolism, appetite, hormones, and digestion. Lastly, the Kapha dosha controls your immune system, strength and stability, muscle growth, and, importantly, weight.

As you can see, these are critical elements to weight loss and keeping them in mind and feeding those three in a positive manner will help to strengthen your body, mind, and spirit and enhance your connectivity with the universe.

Chapter 2: Toxins in the Shadows

You can find it in your water, you can see it in the air you breathe, and if you take merely 30 minutes to Google some of the active and inert ingredients to household cleaners, soaps, or the residue of pesticides on your "fresh" fruits and vegetables, you will be shocked and dismayed—frustrated even. Just because something is labeled "natural," does not necessarily mean that it is healthy. Take corn syrup for example—a sweetener that is prevalent in the United States. It is everywhere, an essential ingredient in every food that even pretends to be sweet. In and of itself and in small amounts, perhaps it isn't horrible, but when you consider the rate at which Americans consume corn syrup, there is no wonder as to why the

States, and other countries, are being overtaken with obesity and health complications therein.

Air pollutants have become so pervasive that cities issue alerts about smog and filth in the air. Many of the pollutants have carcinogenic elements, yet, in big cities, they are almost unavoidable. The problem with pollutants in our air has become so intense that rural areas are being negatively impacted and are discovering the carry-over of these very same pollutants. According to Ayurveda, GMO is very bad and the only solution is to replace the genetically modified organisms with completely natural, organic food.

This is certainly not to say that these pollutants and toxins are placed in our environment intentionally or with malicious intent. In most cases, they are created as a result of someone trying to make our quality of life more palatable. Here is a little experiment for you:

1. Go through all of your kitchen cabinets and look at the labels on your food.

2. Write down all of the words you cannot pronounce.

3. Google them.

4.   Try not to be terrified.

The good news amid all of this horrifying news is that most of these toxins can be eliminated quickly through natural processes such as the one you're learning about in this book—Ayurveda.

There are other toxins coursing through our bodies that are emotional, such as a negative self-image. Toxic thinking produces stress, a loss of joy, and can even lead to clinical depression for some. The reality that can be so elusive is that our happiness goes far beyond just physical appearances, beyond our environment, beyond our sphere of influence, and far beyond what our minds try to convince us.

The fact that you're reading this book right now shows that you have within you unlimited potential and a desire to improve the quality of your life. You're willing to try something that has worked for thousands of years, but it's different and challenging to you and that speaks volumes to your character and the process of eliminating mental and physical toxins from your existence.

When you're detoxifying, you'll be surprised how quickly and easily your unwanted pounds disappear.

Chapter 3: Weight Loss Through Ayurveda Detoxification

When you hear the term "detoxification," our minds within this contemporary culture immediately envision celebrity reality shows where for the first 72 hours of their stay at a rehabilitation facility, they're writhing and screaming in pain and anguish. The microphones and hidden cameras are strategically placed, designed to catch every breathtaking moment of extreme anxiety and suffering. This has been branded into our thinking, unfortunately, because what we're about to discuss is whole different type of detoxification that is actually good for you and doesn't cause pain.

Simply put, imagine a pan of soda in your kitchen sink. When you turn on the tap and the hot water streams into the pan, the water to soda ratio begins to shift. When you apply soap, you'll see some bubbles, perhaps even a fresh, aromatic scent replacing the sugary presence of soda. Eventually, the soda is replaced with water and you have yourself a clean pan. That's what this detoxification represents.

There are two trains of thought in the Ayurvedic community about cleansing, or detoxifying the body. The first dictates a juice-only diet and is certainly not for everyone. In the contemporary culture, most of us have to work, we have to be coherent during most of the day and radical methods of cleansing can be dangerous and unhealthy. The purpose of detoxification is to lead up to a weight loss regimen. The second school of thought (which is what we will follow for the purpose of this book) is much more gradual, less of a shock to the system and does not require absolute fasting.

Consider this the "preparation phase" where you begin to change and adapt your eating habits that will first reduce toxins and then lead you right into the process of losing weight with Ayurveda.

There is a term you need to remember: Ama. Ama is the product of undigested food. It can be a sticky toxic matter that can and most likely will clog the tributaries of your body that bring essential nutrients to your body on a molecular level. In other words, think of it as the difference between 100% and 80/20 fuel (20% being ethanol). While ethanol saves fuel and is from renewable material, it's been known to leave sludge in the fuel system. When there is sludge, fuel can't get to the pistons properly and the aggregate result is that the engine misfires.

Following Ayurveda principles, ama can be caused by impurities stockpiled in the bodies as a result of poor dietary choices, chronic stress, and chemical/pollutants contained in our environments. The accumulation of ama in fat cells forces them to expand, which makes the process of losing weight more difficult. As our bodies age, it is highly recommended to increase detoxification programs.

Your body misfires as well when it is clogged with ama. Here is a list of ama-producing foods that you need to eliminate from your diet immediately.

1. Processed Foods. As delicious as that processed cheese macaroni might taste, it is not worth the lack of energy and the toxins it forces through your veins. Processed meat, processed fruit—all of them are to be avoided at all costs.

2. Pre-packaged Foods. Deli meat in a bag is probably one of the most sodium-laden foods in the universe. The reason it is made in such a way is because with high concentrations of sodium and chemicals, the product can sit on the shelves for longer periods of time.

3. Heavy Dairy. Hard cheese, even cheddar cheese, has high concentrations of fat that can be far from healthy for your arteries and coronary health.

4. Yogurt. Even though some preach the probiotic salvation of yogurt, it too contains heavy carbohydrates and fat.

5. Yeast. Bread is a delicious, tempting, palate-pleasing delight for most of us, however, it is loaded with carbohydrates and believe it or not, is tough to ingest.

Now that we have covered a few of the ama-producing foods, let's consider the foods that will reduce the amount of ama your body produces.

1.   Fresh Fruit. Juicy fruits are great cleansers— such as cooked prunes or figs during breakfast with an apple.

2.   Leafy Vegetables. You've heard it said that leafy greens are the way to go where nutrition delivery systems are concerned. Cabbage (fresh) or even Brussels sprouts are good alternatives— but you can't load them up with cheeses and heavy butter.

3.   Spices. While spices may not be a staple of your diet, there are spices that can help to open up the vessels in the body. Tumeric, coriander, fenugreek, fennel, and ginger are exceptional at flushing toxins in the skin, the colon, the liver, and even the urinary tract.

4. Grains, Grains, Grains. Light grains like barley, small servings of rice, quinoa, and oats are good for the digestive system and amazingly helpful in flushing toxins from your body.

As odd and unusual as it may seem, warm drinking water helps with flushing toxins from the body. If you so choose, you can add some of the spices mentioned above (3) for flavor and additional detoxifying qualities.

The Ayurveda way of detoxifying encourages a reduction (if not elimination) of all meats from your diet, however, it is understood that it may be very difficult for some, therefore, if you're going to eat meat, ensure that it is extra lean and void of chemicals.

There may come a time when you reintroduce the foods you're used to (with the exception of the foods mentioned earlier in the chapter), but you will do so in very gradual, very small amounts. What you're going to learn next will be the Ayurveda way for weight loss and as you begin to see results, you may not want to ever go back to the eating habits you followed previously.

Chapter 4: Ayurveda Weight Loss Plan

As you can see thus far, there is more to Ayurveda than a few changes in food intake. Ayurveda brings you to a place where your system is more in tune with the universe and focuses your mind, body, and spirit on the connectivity therein. Through the detoxification process, you will no doubt already begin seeing changes in your energy level, the efficiency of your digestive tract, and maybe notice you lost a couple pounds. The detox aspect of Ayurveda is like the doorway to healthy weight loss, and now, we are going to walk through the door.

In this next phase of Ayurveda weight loss, you are going to challenge your senses, break old habits, and learn to meditate on your goals and your whole being—not just your body. To begin with, here are a few suggestions to kick off the weight loss plan:

1.   Meditation. Find yourself a quiet place every morning and spend 15 minutes with your eyes closed, concentrating on the whole body. Think of what your body is feeling, allow no constraints on your mind, and allow your spirit to reach out to the world around you. Get yourself into the habit of meditation, at the very least, five days a week.

2.   Exercise. Ayurveda does not require a gym membership, or that you attempt to go on the body building circuit. Any type of physical exertion that raises your heart rate and makes you sweat is perfectly fine.

3.   Warm Lemon Water. You read that right— with your breakfast, before your coffee, drink a 300 ml glass of warm lemon water to kick start the digestive system and improve "movement," as it were. Never, under any circumstances should you use a microwave oven to warm or heat water. After you have consumed the warm lemon water, give yourself 10–15 minutes before eating or

drinking any other foods. Microwave ovens create a Vata imbalance which results in increased ama production.

4. Stick to Three. You're breaking habits and changing your lifestyle. Snacking between meals is no longer an acceptable practice. The temptations, the cravings may come along but that's when you use your meditation and focused breathing to remind yourself of your goals and where you desire to see yourself.

5. Expand the Tastes. Ayurveda recognizes a total of six tastes. They include: salty, bitter, sour, pungent, sweet, and astringent. Explore each of the different tastes using organically grown produce and fruits. Sodium and high concentrations of fat in much of the diet within the Western culture is part of the epidemic of obesity. Ayurveda encourages expansion of the taste buds, to experience the whole spectrum of flavors on a regular basis—not to focus on one or two, but all of them.

6. Sun, Sun. Go to bed at sunset, awaken to the sunrise. For centuries prior to the age of technology, our forefathers (and mothers) had absolutely no reason to stay up—television, Netflix, and the like weren't around and unless it was a

night of religious celebration, the farmers and craftsmen of the day went to bed at a decent time (with the sunset) and awakened early (sunrise).

7. Move It, Move It. You've just consumed an Ayurveda-recommended meal of organic fruits, grains, and vegetables, now what? The old habits may have been to plop down on the couch or in the recliner to sleep it off and focus brain power on the television. Not any longer. Get up, move around and get some exercise after a meal. We're not talking about running a marathon or loading up at the gym—just a light walk with the family will suffice.

8. Switch It Up.   Normally, we have a light breakfast, average lunch, and we chow down for dinner. With Ayurveda, you're going to switch that up quite a bit. Your largest meal by far will be your lunchtime meal. Your dinner will be more like your lunch has been in days gone by, and your breakfast will be loaded with healthy sugars and carbohydrates but lighter than the biscuits and gravy you have been used to.

9. Yoga can be an excellent tool within the Ayurveda plan to help with weight loss. Stretching, elongating muscle tissue is part of

yoga. Ayurveda highly recommends adding yoga to your weight loss plan.

10. Avoid the Cold. During your detoxification and weight loss program, avoid cold food or cold water with your meal.

11. Tea for Two. Throughout the day, sip warm tea between your regularly scheduled meals. This will help increase the fire in your metabolic system that will melt fat and detoxify your body.

Those eleven simple steps in the Ayurveda ladder will go a long way to breaking bad habits and developing new, healthy ones. It is important to note that Ayurveda is not designed to be rigid, forceful or dogmatic—those impulses are not healthy and often lead to increased stress which, in turn, encourages one to rediscover bad habits. Ayurveda is forgiving, fluid, and natural and nowhere in that process is there to be any element that increases your stress or anxiety levels.

Remember the three doshas we discovered in the last chapter? This is where we learn how critical they are in the workings of Ayurveda. These three doshas are core metabolic attributes that give us a very clear indication as to our body types and what types of diet we should pursue:

Hyper Dosha	Attributes	Diet
Kapha dry, & light	Cold, wet, & heavy	Warm,
Pitta & heavy	Hot, wet, & light	Cool, dry,
Vata	Cold, dry, & light	Warm, moist & heavy

If you're concerned about which dosha is overactive in your system, there are quite a few locations online where you can answer survey questions about your body, your mind, your habits, and your motivation. These surveys will help you to identify which of the doshas are predominant to you naturally, and which may be overactive and causing problems.

Here are some facts that Ayurveda has taught for thousands of years.

a.   The body naturally craves what it needs during the accompanying season. During the winter months, the body craves heavier meals to prepare for the cold temperatures. During the summer months, the body is in cool-down mode and craves fruits and vegetables that are fresh and light.

b.   Moderation is key. Alcohol is not evil in and of itself, however, if it is consumed in an overabundance, the damage to the liver is irreparable and the body fat index increases. A glass of wine, however, is not bad for the system at all and in some cases, can help the body in the digestive phase.

c.   Teamwork. Having an accountability partner is not a bad thing at all. Though you and you alone are responsible for your happiness and balance with your environment, an encouraging word or smiling face can go a long way to helping you reach your goals.

d.   Balance. Not only are you trying to lose weight and develop a healthy lifestyle, but Ayurveda strives to bring your whole being into balance with itself and in so doing, bring a balance between you and the environment— the spirit, the essence of our universe—around you.

e.   It's a marathon, not a sprint. After your time of Ayurveda cleansing and implementing the diet changes, you will see a change in weight, attitude, strength, and endurance.   Every person is different, comprised of different elements and therefore, the results will vary with each individual. You are to remember that this is a long-term lifestyle change and there will be peaks and valleys. Using the Ayurveda methods of spices, moments of meditation and concentration on the wholeness of the being, the valleys will be much more shallow and easier to be traveled.

f. Don't forget the herbs. Ayurvedic herbs are not difficult to find either online or at your local health food store. In the second chapter, we provided you with an abbreviated list of helpful Ayurvedic herbs to use in weight loss as well as the cleansing. There is, however, a formula of Ayurvedic herbs that is effective to all people, regardless of the dosha of an individual. Start with 500mg of puskarmool, amla (Indian gooseberry), nagarmotha (nut grass), kutki, powdered tumeric, and vacha. 125mg of black pepper, long pepper, and daruhirdra. Taken daily, this formula will aid in the process of healthy weight loss.

g. Triphala trifecta. Triphala literally means "three fruits" and is widely used for the purposes of immune systems, improving digestion, mild laxative, diabetic aid, and gastrointestinal cleansing. The three dried and powdered fruits are: Amalaki (Indian gooseberry), Bibhitaki

(Beleric), and Haritaki (inknut). Triphala is a potent, yet safe Ayurvedic that has been reported to help with weight loss because of the improvement made in the digestive system which increases metabolism.

With all of these factors in mind, let's consider what your average work day would be:

1.   Rise at sunrise. It may take a little bit of time to get used to the alternate sleep patterns, so be prepared to be tired for the first few weeks of your Ayurveda trek.

2.   Warm glass of lemon water (freshly squeezed, not artificial flavoring).

3.   Meditation. 10 to 15 minutes of meditation, focusing on wholeness of your body, mind, and spirit and connectivity to the universe around you. Allow the meditation time to charge your proverbial batteries, prepare you for the day and strengthen your resolve to continue down that road of healthy life choices resulting in weight loss.

4.   Brief exercise. Spend 30 minutes doing exercise, enough to bring up a sweat. How you

exercise is less important than the fact that you ARE exercising.

5.   Eat a fruit combination for breakfast, ensuring that you consume the fruits that are in season at that time.   Apples, figs, pears, or prunes are excellent choices for a morning meal.

6.   Shower, go about your day until...

7.   Lunch.   Remember—this will be the largest meal of the day and you should have a good mixture of proteins and carbohydrates. Top off with a warm glass of water accompanied by one of the Ayurvedic spices mentioned previously.

8.   Work until it's time to go home.

9.   Eat a light dinner.   This will include your triphala, protein, fresh fruit, and fresh, organic vegetables.   This meal is designed to give you the much needed nutrients for the evening and help you sleep soundly.

10. Walk off that meal.   This would be a perfect time for family and doing something that requires movement together.   Go for a walk or a brief jog, and enjoy your time with the family and put your mind into a thankful mode.

11. Bed at sunset. As the sun goes down, your peace and tranquility rises. A good night's rest can be as therapeutic in the Ayurvedic system and breathing. Sleep reduces stress, anxiety and repairs muscle tissue for the next day.

Clearly, this represents a radical change in your diet, your attitude, and a collective unity of your body, mind, and spirit. That wholeness, that unity if you will, will bring you closer in tune with the world around you and when that happens, you will improve your health and lose significant weight. The beauty of it all is that you're doing it in a healthy, natural way without the aid of dangerous pharmaceuticals or fad diets.

Chapter 5: Lifestyle Choices

Following the Ayurveda methods is a radical departure from "normalcy" for many individuals. The change in sleep patterns, the adjustment in dietary requirements, the mental awareness of body, mind, and spirit. It's not an easy process and requires an enormous amount of commitment, dedication, and help from loved ones. These lifestyle choices are going to be uncomfortable, however, Ayurveda has built-in processes and methods to deal with the stress and anxiety of making radical changes.

First, there is an inherent human desire to take a path of least resistance. Ayurveda's meditation element, coupled with the dietary supplements and natural herbs will help overcome the temptation to quit.

Second, consuming lemon water in the morning will serve to get your system going and hydrate the body. One of the biggest causes for loss of energy is that of hydration. Ayurveda encourages the consumption of water with herbs or juice to maintain hydration.

Third, changing sleep patterns in the Ayurveda method becomes natural and abundantly clear that you've been missing out on solid, peaceful sleep. The human existence from the dawn of time has followed solar and lunar schedules for sleep and work. Ayurveda encourages the same patterns in a contemporary setting.

Fourth, there will be naysayers. We all know the types—the individuals who are emotional vampires, sucking the joy out of life. When you're following the Ayurvedic weight loss method, those who are negative stand out as individuals who are to be avoided and ignored. As your awareness and wholeness grows, you will easily be able to identify those around you who are struggling with their wholeness.

Fifth, "lifestyle" means long term. Ayurveda has been practiced for 5,000 years and nowhere throughout its history has there been a short-term fix, but rather a dedication to lifestyle changes that are healthier, more balanced with the seasons, and unifies the person with the universe around him or her.

Sixth, Ayurveda is gender-neutral and non-judgmental. Regardless of gender, regardless of sexual preference, regardless of religious affiliations, Ayurveda is designed to accommodate and welcome any who choose to accept the unification of the mind, body, and spirit.

Seventh, becoming aware and in tune with your emotions rather than suppressing them will help reduce stress, anxiety, increase the metabolism, and improve the overall outlook and attitude of the participant in Ayurveda. Ayurveda is inclusive of emotional awareness and not exclusionary.

Eighth, bonding with your natural surroundings will bring a sense of peace and tranquility and help in the alignment of the whole person. Ayurveda teaches that we are all a part of the universal consciousness, therefore, we should enjoy creation for what it is as it brings us closer to the unified whole.

One of the most difficult lifestyle changes in Ayurveda is the dramatic reduction of meat consumption and an awareness of the benefits of fresh fruits and vegetables as well as legumes for proteins. The body contains a plethora of toxins that were consumed by previous eating patterns and with the Ayurvedic method, those toxins are driven out of the system and replaced with wholesome, essential nutrients. Breaking the habit of fatty foods can be a remarkably difficult task, yet as you have seen, Ayurveda provides built-in stop gaps for even the worst withdrawal.

One of the most overlooked aspects of the human battle against obesity and all of the diseases that come along with weight gain is diabetes. While diabetes can be genetic, it is also developed by long standing habits of consumption of sweets and carbohydrates in overabundance. Diabetes can be a killer. It leads to liver failure, pancreatic cancer, mood swings, makes wounds and injuries slower to heal, and increases the risk of cardiovascular disease. Ayurveda, just by the very nature of the dietary requirements, fights against the possibility of diabetes and if diabetes is already present, Ayurveda can bring the blood sugars into balance.

Ayurveda is a lifestyle choice—a positive choice that will bring better physical, emotional and physical health.

Conclusion

Thank you again for purchasing Ayurveda Weight Loss: The Ultimate Guide to Successful Ayurvedic Detox and Weight Loss!

I hope this book was able to help you to understand the many great benefits of Ayurveda as a weight loss method. As you have read, it transcends just a couple hours at the gym each week, but rather approaches the problem of excess weight with a whole-being method. Ayurveda seeks to bring together the mind, body, and spirit of the participant and to do so in a healthy, natural method rather than depending upon pharmaceuticals and fad diet schemes.

The next step is to contact your family practice physician and schedule an appointment to discuss your body's needs during the Ayurveda process. Your physician will tell you whether or not your body is in a condition to make this incredible life change.

After your cleansing period, you will start on your diet regimen and watch the weight fall off as your health improves and your spiritual oneness with the creation becomes intensified.

Then, share it with your family and friends. Encourage them to do that which you've done and make it a family affair.

Finally, if you enjoyed this book, then I'd like to ask you for a favor. Would you be kind enough to leave a review for this book on Amazon? It'd be greatly appreciated!

Thank you and good luck!

Other books by Michael Cesar:

Tantric Love —The Sacred Union Of Souls

Improve Your Love Life And Your Relationship with Tantra—By Michael Cesar

The union of two people on more than a physical level is the ultimate goal as you read through this book. Once you allow yourself to be one with your partner and the divine, you will experience true sexual freedom and lose your inhibitions with your partner.

Success Habits

Kaizen — Improve Your Life and Become Successful by Taking One Small Step at a Time — By Michael Cesar

This book is a dynamic resource for men and women alike to set small, attainable goals that are measurable and maintain a pattern of positive behavior. "Kaizen" means "change for better," and is created to increase your productivity at work as well as at home.

Effortless Manifestation Magic And Miracles

Discover The Single Most Powerful Method Of Manifesting Your Dream Life From Oneness - By Michael Cesar

Within the universe lays a wealth of information that the human mind has only just begun to tap into. Manifesting is one of those sources which are readily available to anyone who seeks to obtain the miracles that the universe is waiting to impart on every individual. Similar to prayer and meditation, manifesting is a personal journey into the magic of self-discovery and a unique oneness with the world around us.

Ayurveda Weight Loss

The Ultimate Guide to Successful Ayurvedic Detox and Weight Loss —By Michael Cesar

This book covers the cleansing/detoxification process, the Ayurvedic diet, the lifestyle changes, as well as tips and aids for daily life and maintaining commitment to your weight loss goals and personal goals.

The Natural Cure for Erectile Dysfunction

How to Cure Erectile Dysfunction And Impotency Permanently In The Comfort of your own Home By Following These Simple And Easy Proven Methods—By Michael Cesar

Discover how to finally overcome Erectile Dysfunction, impotency, premature ejaculation, inhibited ejaculation, sexual inexperience, pornography addictions, or sexual addiction as well as other sexual issues.